D1391771

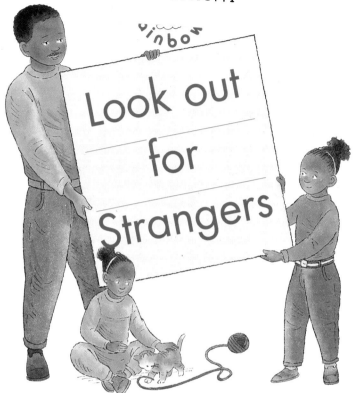

rainbow

Look out
for
Strangers

Paul Humphrey and
Alex Ramsay

Illustrated by
Colin King

Evans

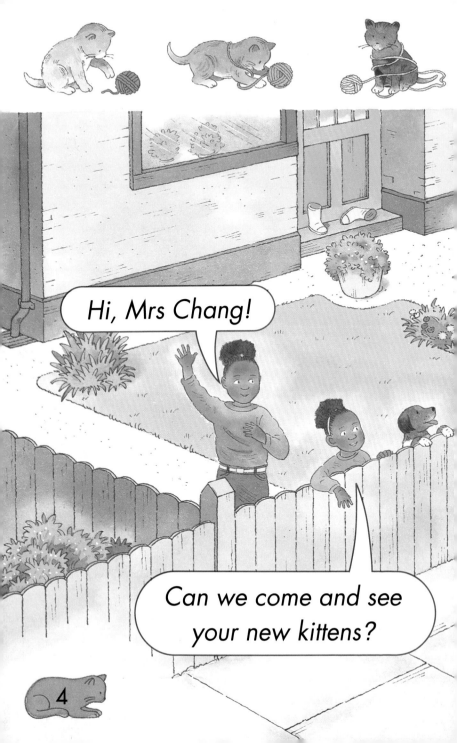

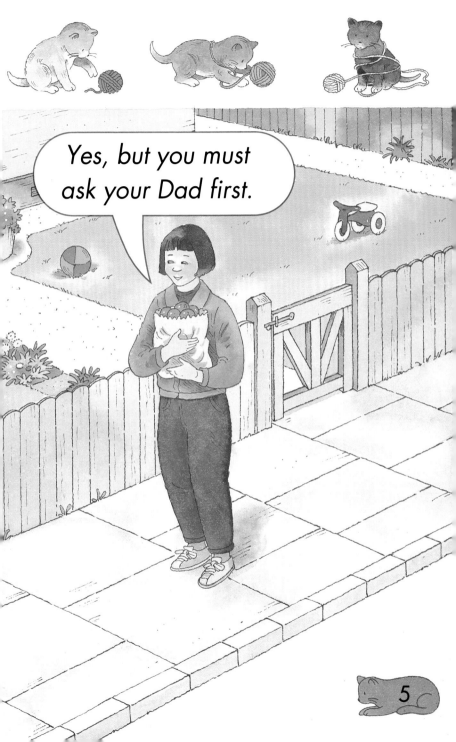

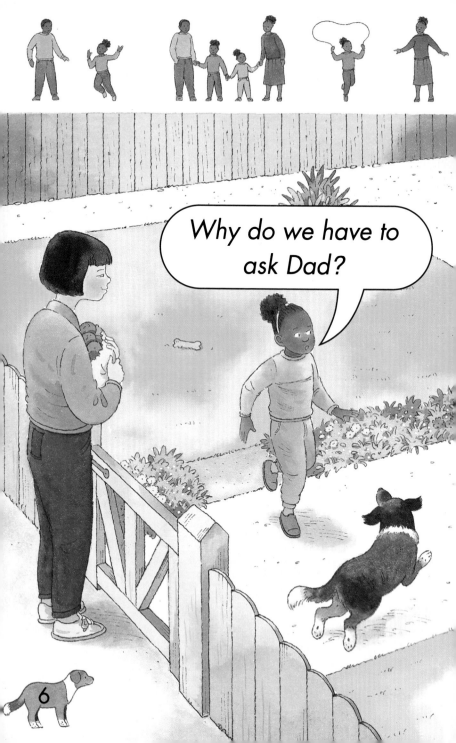

6

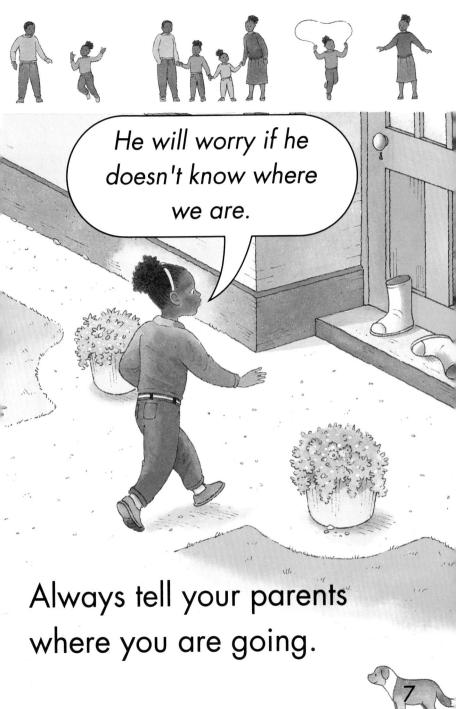

Always tell your parents
where you are going.

7

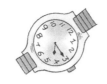

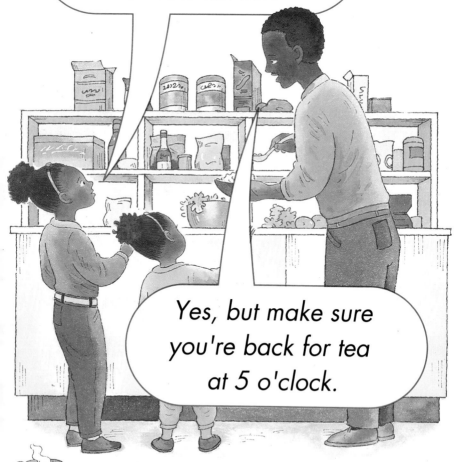

Mum or Dad must know what time you are coming home.

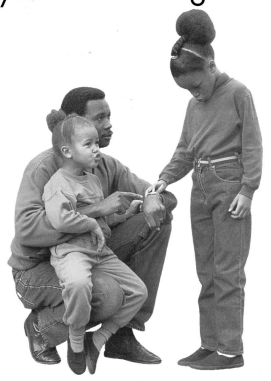

Then they can come and find you if they are worried.

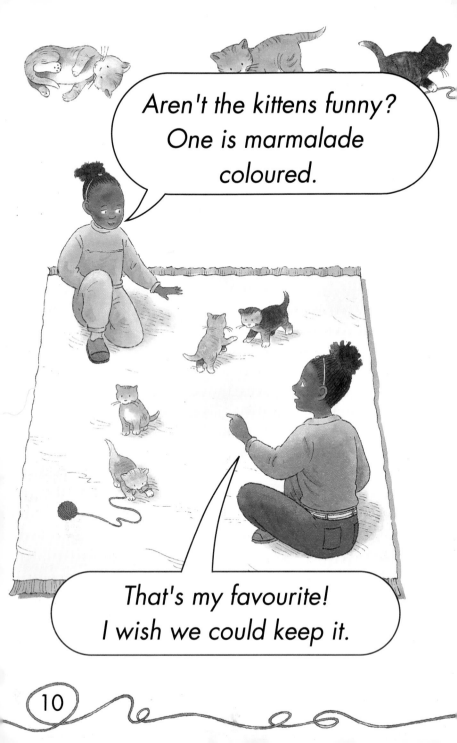

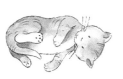
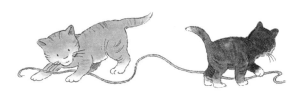

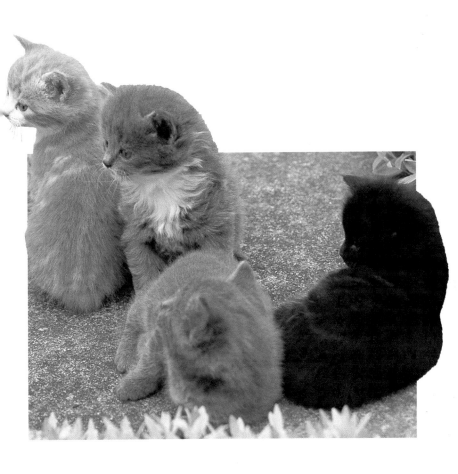

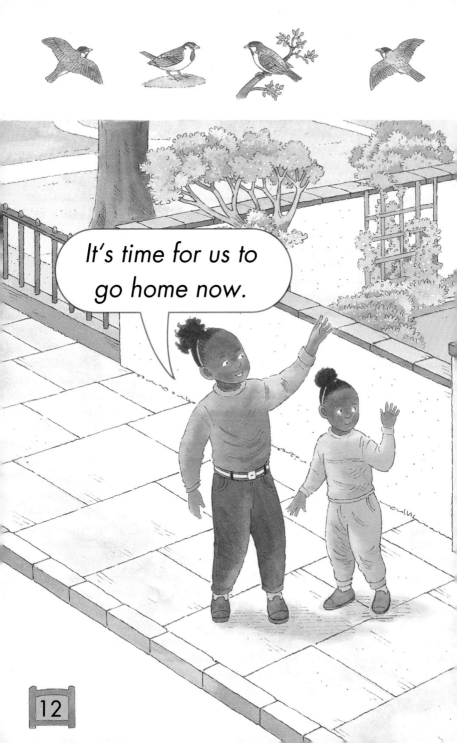

It's time for us to go home now.

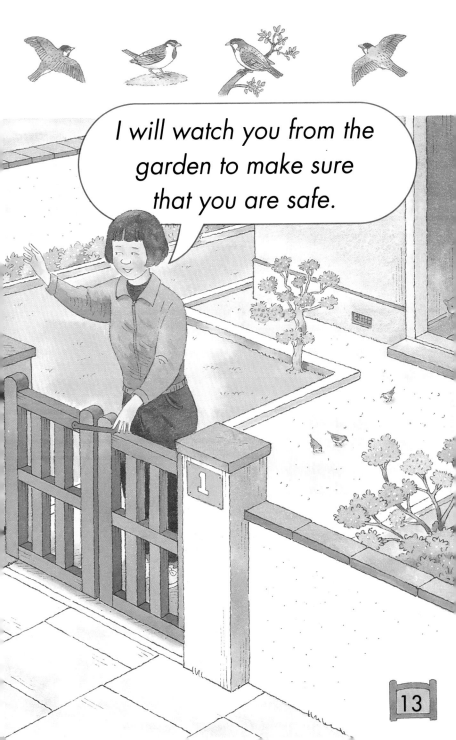

13

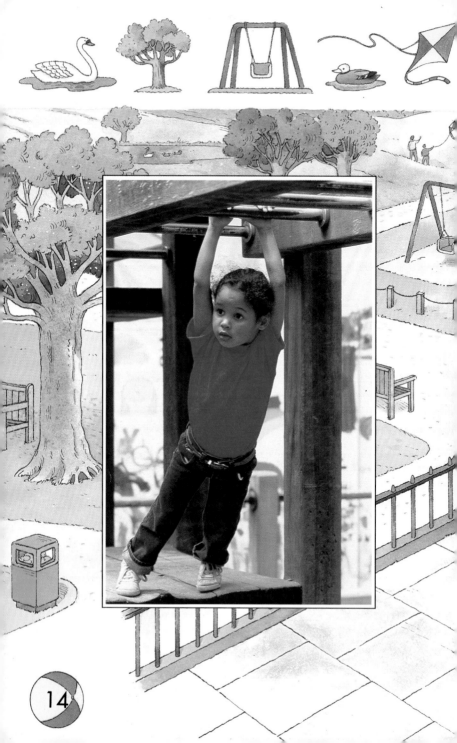

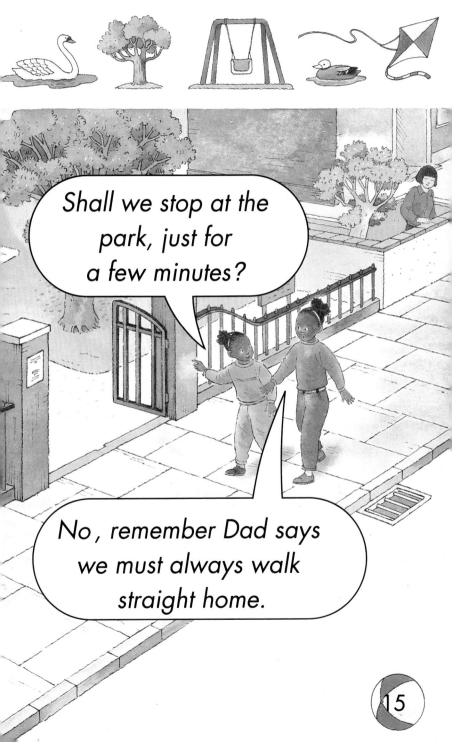

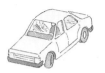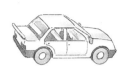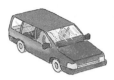

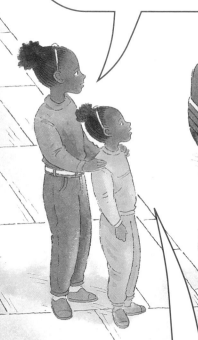

Look, there are Dad's friends Mr and Mrs Adams in their new car.

Hello, can we give you a lift somewhere?

No, thank you, Dad is waiting for us.

16

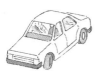 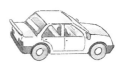 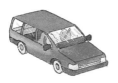

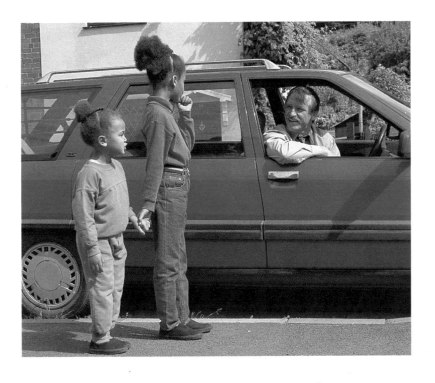

Never get in a car with someone, even if you know them, without asking Mum or Dad first.

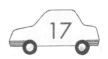

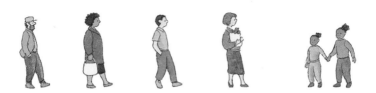

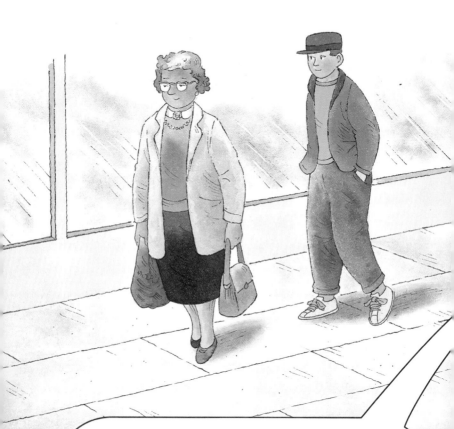

My teacher says that some grown-ups who look nice are unkind to children.

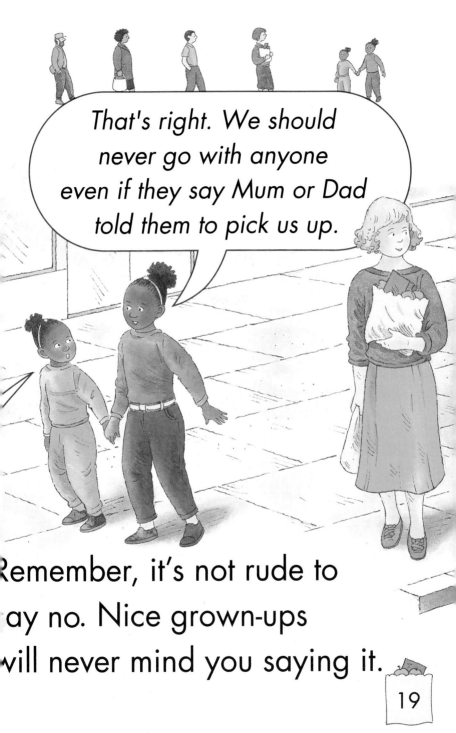

That's right. We should never go with anyone even if they say Mum or Dad told them to pick us up.

Remember, it's not rude to say no. Nice grown-ups will never mind you saying it.

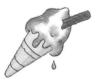

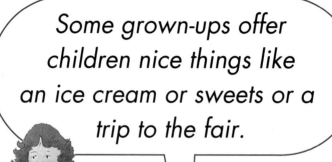

Some grown-ups offer children nice things like an ice cream or sweets or a trip to the fair.

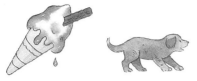

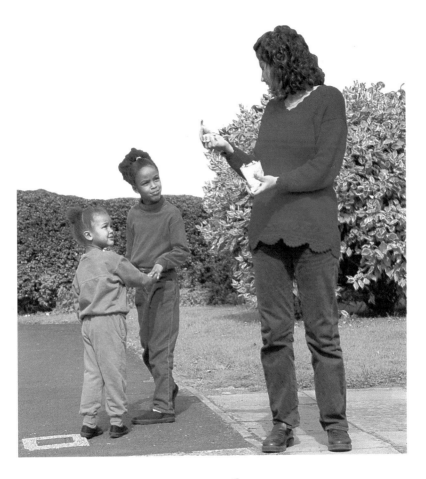

Always say no if a stranger offers you treats.

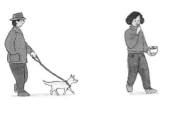

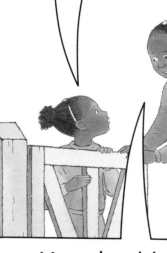

If a stranger offered me sweets I would say no thank you.

You should always tell someone about it, too.

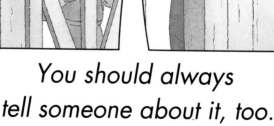

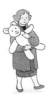

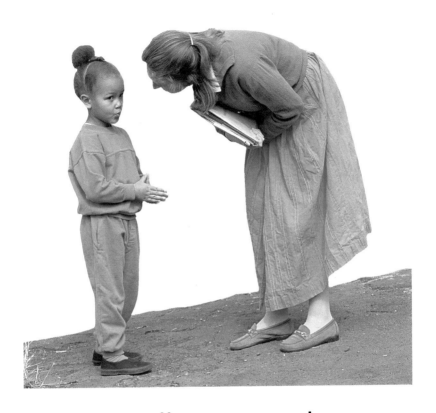

You can tell your teacher,
your parents or grandparents
or a police officer.

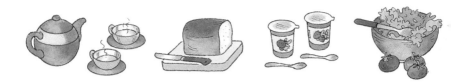

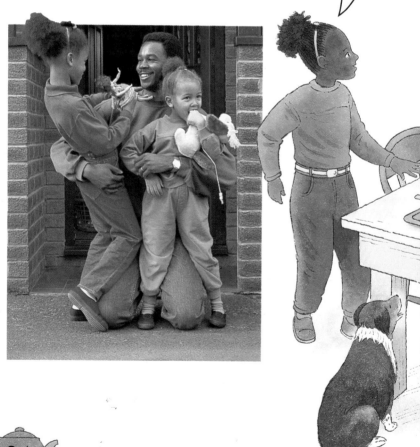

Look we're just in time for tea!

24

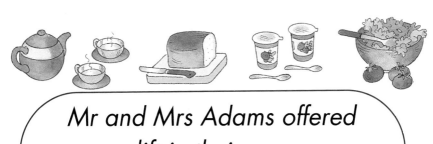

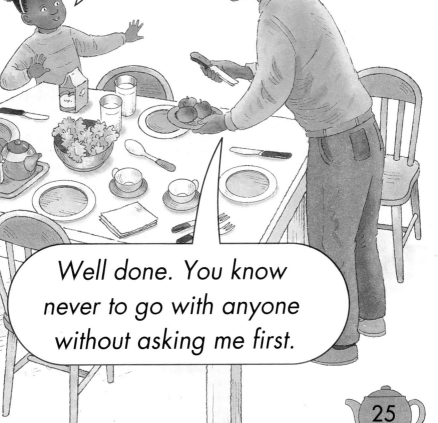

Mr and Mrs Adams offered us a lift in their new car, but we said no.

Well done. You know never to go with anyone without asking me first.

25

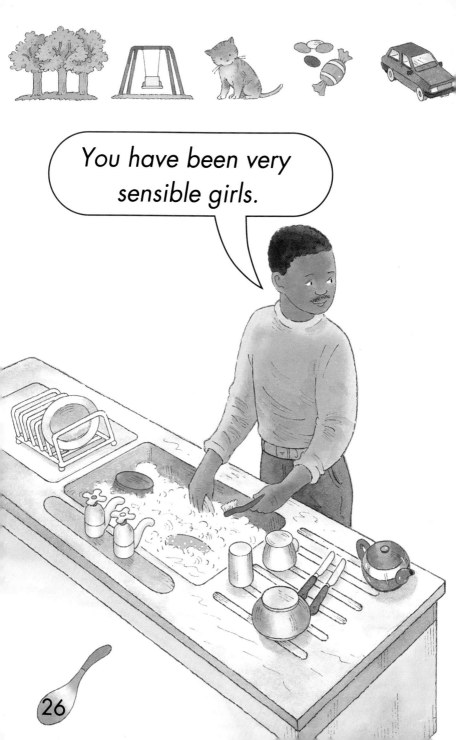

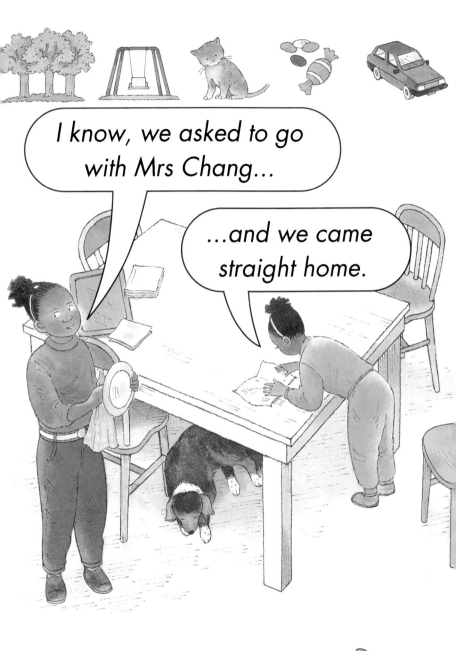

27

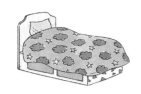
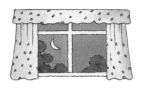

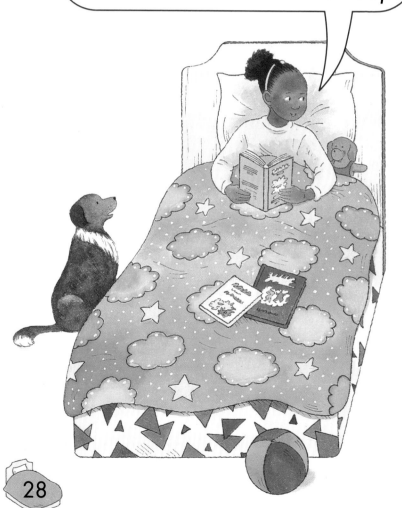

Mrs Chang said we could have one of the kittens to keep.

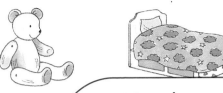
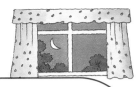
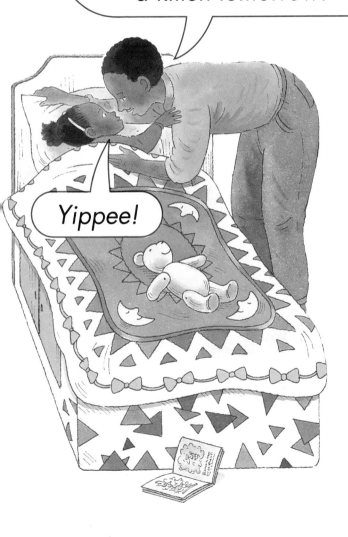

29

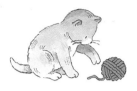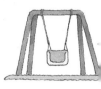

Some rules to remember:

1. Make sure your Mum or Dad knows where you are (see pages **6 - 8**).

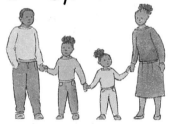

2. Make sure Mum or Dad knows when you are coming home (see pages **8 - 9**).

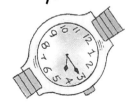

30